Neha Nilesh Lavhade

Ergonomics

Neha Nilesh Lavhade

Ergonomics

LAP LAMBERT Academic Publishing

Cover image: www.ingimage.com

Publisher:
LAP LAMBERT Academic Publishing
is a trademark of
Dodo Books Indian Ocean Ltd. and OmniScriptum S.R.L publishing group

120 High Road, East Finchley, London, N2 9ED, United Kingdom
Str. Armeneasca 28/1, office 1, Chisinau MD-2012, Republic of Moldova, Europe
Managing Directors: Ieva Konstantinova, Victoria Ursu
info@omniscriptum.com

Printed at: see last page
ISBN: 978-620-8-43998-9

ERGONOMICS

Dr. Neha Nilesh Lavhade

Content:

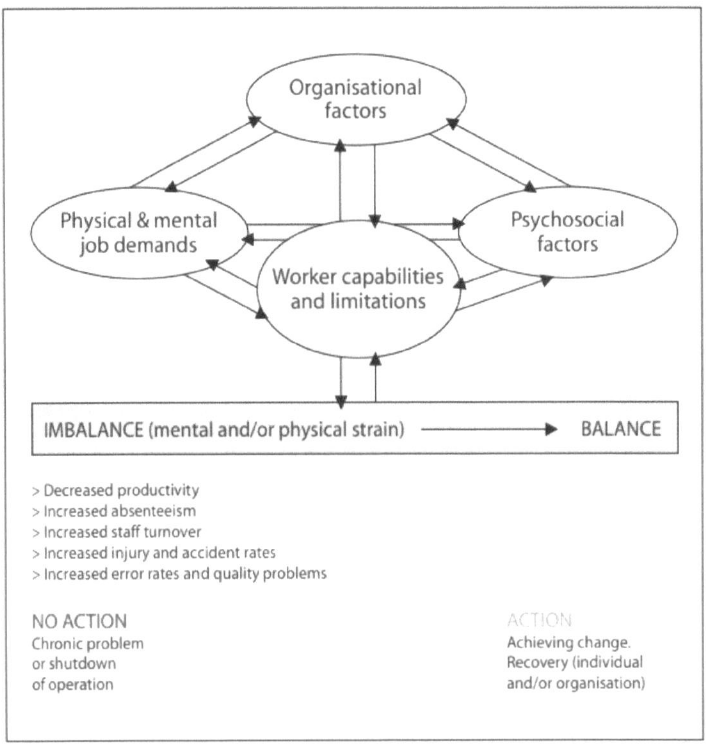

Figure 1 Physical, mental and psychosocial factors influencing workers' health.
From Aickin, Lusted and McPhee 2009

- **Introduction:**

- Derived from the Greek ergon (work) and nomos (laws) to denote the science of work, ergonomics is a systems-oriented discipline that extends across all aspects of human activity, and therefore promotes a holistic approach to enhancing the well-being of people at work.
- To achieve this it considers the physical, cognitive, social, organisational and environmental aspects of work and the impact, both positive and negative, that these may have on the worker.
- Practicing Ergonomists must have a broad understanding of the full scope of the discipline and be able to apply the principles in practice to improve working conditions.
- An ergonomic process or program uses the principles of a safety and health program to address and reduce ergonomic risk factors such as forceful exertion, awkward postures, contact stress, repetitive movements, and vibration. Some examples include frequently lifting heavy items, awkward bending, frequently reaching overhead or working with the hands above head height, frequently pushing/pulling/carrying heavy loads, working in squatting or kneeling postures, using tools while wrist is significantly bent, performing the same similar tasks repetitively several times a minute, using fingers, palms, or hands to press or insert parts with high force, sustained or static postures or positions; and using vibrating tools or tools that press into the muscles or nerves.
- Routine exposure to these ergonomic risk factors for several hours a day can cause soft tissue injuries or musculoskeletal disorders (MSDs).
- Some examples of MSDs include carpal tunnel syndrome, tendinitis, rotator cuff injuries, muscle strains, and low back injuries, as well as other disorders to muscles, nerves, blood vessels, ligaments, and tendons.
- Working in cold temperatures can aggravate MSDs. An ergonomic process or program with employee participation helps identify hazards and improvements to lessen muscle fatigue, reduce medical costs and days away from work, increase productivity, and reduce the number and severity of work-related MSDs.
- Ergonomics is balancing the task demands and work capacity. The two factors must be balanced to achieve high work performance. Poor balance between task demands and work capacity will adversely affect the work system or the worker. One of the

negative impacts caused is fatigue. Fatigue will not only affect workers physically and mentally but also decreases productivity levels. Low workers' productivity will harm the company economically and will affect the workers' welfare.

- **What is ergonomics?**

1. "Ergonomics is the scientific discipline concerned with the fundamental understanding of interactions among humans and other elements of a system, and the profession that applies theory, principles, data and methods to design in order to optimise human well-being and overall system performance" (International Ergonomics Association (IEA), 2000).
2. According to Nurmianto (1996), ergonomics is a study of the system in which humans, work facilities, and the environment interact with the main purpose of adjusting the working atmosphere with human beings.
3. Tarwaka and Sudiajeng (2004) defined ergonomics as the performance or the ability of a human depends on the comparison between the size of the work demands on the large ability of the worker, when:
   • Task demands exceeding the workers' ability or capacity can cause overstress, accidents, fatigue, injury, illness, pain and others
   • Task demands much lower than the workers' ability will result in under-stress and boredom
   • Balanced task demand will enable a comfortable condition, safe and productive.

Ergonomics Domains of Specialization:

According to the International Ergonomics Association, there are three broad domains of ergonomics:

- Physical
- Cognitive
- Organizational

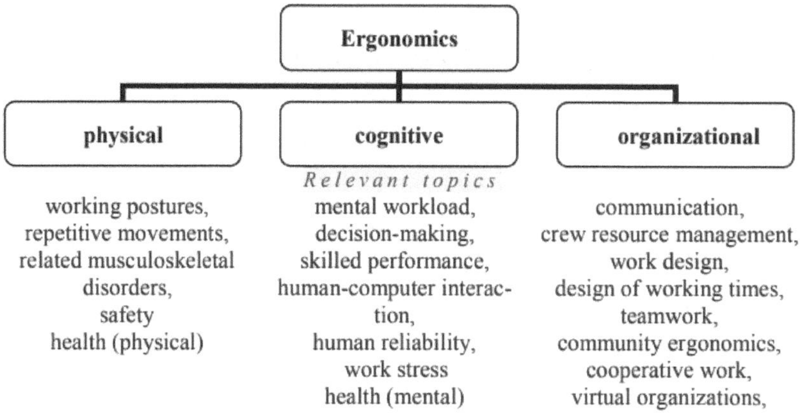

Physical ergonomics

It is concerned with human anatomical, anthropometric, physiological and biomechanical characteristics as they relate to physical activity. Relevant topics include working postures, materials handling, repetitive movements, heavy work, work-related Musculo skeletal disorders, workplace layout ,noise, thermal conditions and vibration ,safety and health, as these relate to work.

Cognitive Ergonomics

Cognitive ergonomics is concerned with mental processes, such as perception, memory, reasoning, and motor response, as they affect interactions among humans and other elements of a system. Relevant topics include mental workload, decision-making, skilled performance, human-computer interaction, human error, work stress and training as these may relate to the way humans work in systems.

Organizational Ergonomics

Organizational ergonomics is concerned with the optimization of sociotechnical systems, including their organizational structures, policies, and processes. Relevant topics include human system considerations in communication, human resource management, work design, design of work schedules, team work, participatory design, community ergonomics, cooperative work, new work models, virtual organisations, tele-work and quality management.

Classification of ergonomics - Karsh et al, 2014:

1. **Macro Ergonomics**

   Macro ergonomics is the activity of analysing work postures, estimating productivity, designing work tools. Macro ergonomics has several studies including the structural dimensions of the work system. Macro ergonomics is more broadly ergonomic and needs to be implemented through integration into a larger environment (corporate organization) known as macro ergonomics, which places the production system as a work organization. In subsequent developments, the work system design approach is associated with organizational structure, human and organizational interaction and motivational aspects of the work. This approach is known as Macro Ergonomic. In industrial systems, this approach is also called Organizational Design (OD) and is used in the design of organizational structures and relationships among components of such structures. Hendrick (2002) said there are three sequential generation of ergonomic development which focused on :

   • designing specific tasks, working groups, human-machinery relationships, including displays, workplace settings, the physical environment of work. It is directed at anthropometry and human physical characteristics and their implications in product design.

   • cognitive factors reflected in the design of the system. The emphasized development model is user-system interface technology. The ergonomic development basis started to touch many problems of technology systems. This approach is called the human factor engineering or cognitive ergonomics.

   • focusing on Organizational Ergonomics, such as macro system design, work system optimization in relation to organizational behaviour and organizational psychology. The emphasized development model is organization machine interface technology. Assessment of the organization was from top to bottom using the sociotechnical system approach.

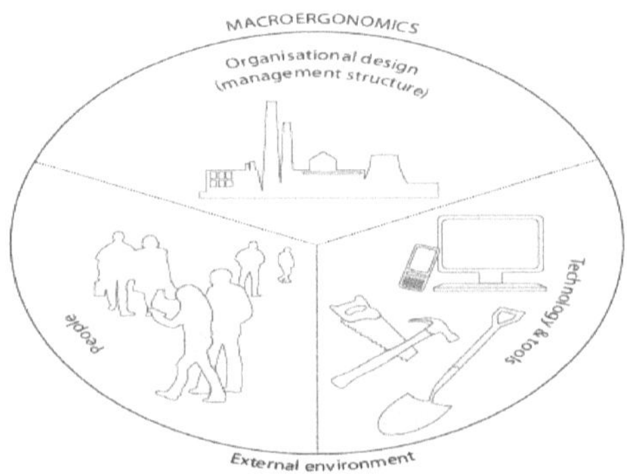

2. Micro Ergonomics

Ergonomics can be regarded as ergonomics in small scope or traditional ergonomics. Activities analysing work or worker posture, estimating productivity, designing work tools, work physiology, work biomechanics, physical environment, anthropometry, percentiles, standard time and others, these are scientific within the scope of micro ergonomics. Thus, micro ergonomics is an ergonomic approach to a process aimed specifically at a specific process. In the early development of ergonomics, the ergonomic is more focused on the design of work systems that emphasize on the relevance of the suitability of human capabilities with work /tasks that must be completed. Such an approach is characteristic of micro ergonomics. The current development of science sees that ergonomic assessment is not only necessary and micro analysed.

Much of ergonomics has focused on people working with tools, machines and other equipment. This is what we call the "human-machine" interface and is now often referred to as micro ergonomics. Any incompatibility between task requirements and the capabilities (mental and/or physical) of the worker can result in a sub-optimal situation. In turn, this may lead to errors, accidents and injuries. Working with employees Ergonomists can identify and prioritise problem areas and propose possible solutions. If necessary, they may recommend a redesign of the workplace, the tasks and/or the organisation of the work to accommodate individual workers as well as groups of workers.

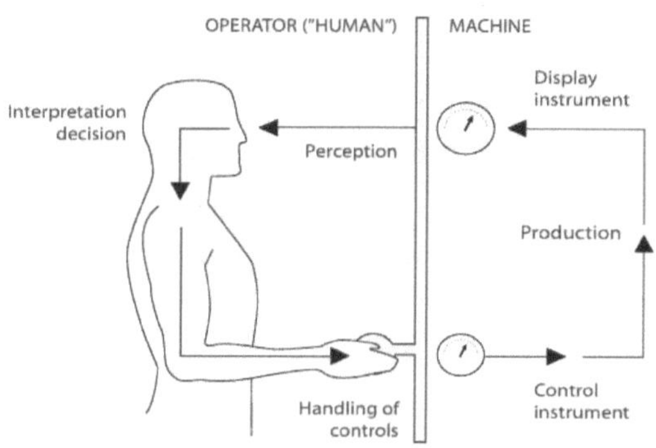

3. Meso Ergonomics

Meso ergonomics is in-between micro and macro ergonomics. However, the boundaries are unknown. Meso ergonomics encompasses relationships between individuals and organizations and sociotechnical systems. In designing the work system, the main factor to be considered as the centre of attention is the human factor. The approach in industrial design is Human Integrated Design, that utilises all information about human beings covering its advantages and disadvantages and being integrated as the basis for a system design.

Principles of ergonomics:

1. Work in a neutral position.

Whether you work sitting or standing and moving throughout the day, it's important to keep your body in a neutral posture. There are several areas of the body that this principle commonly affects. The first is the back. A healthy spine follows an S-curve, and it's important to maintain this curve while working to avoid strain on your back. If you work in a seated position, good lumbar support is key. For those who stand or move around a facility, it can be helpful to place one foot up on a footrest when standing still, and when you need to lift something, make sure you lift from your legs rather than from your back.

Other areas of the body that may be out of alignment are the neck, elbows, and wrists. To reduce strain on these areas and keep them in alignment, try adjusting your equipment or work position to keep your muscles in a more relaxed position.

2. Decrease the need for excessive force.

Imagine a time when you had to use your full body weight to move an object. That's what this principle is referring to. Pushing, pulling, and lifting heavy items can strain your joints, creating the potential for fatigue or injury. Rather than using excessive force, try to identify tools or strategies that can lighten the load you need to move. It may be as simple as using a cart or hoist to move heavy items, or you may need to make changes to your workflow to lessen the distance you need to travel or the number of items you need to transport.

3. Keep materials within easy reach.

Try extending your arms and outlining a semicircle in front of you. This is your reach envelope, and items you use frequently should be inside this semicircle at your workstation. To accommodate your reach envelope, you may need to rearrange your area so you're no longer reaching for frequently used items. Adjusting your seat and armrests can also bring things like machine controls within reach to reduce fatigue. This principle also applies when reaching into boxes or bins. Rather than straining your shoulders to reach higher, simply tilt the box or place it on a lower surface before reaching inside.

4. Work at the proper height.

Having a work surface that's too high or too low can strain the back, neck, and shoulders. Most routine work should be done at elbow height whether you're sitting or standing. However, if you work with heavy tools, you may want to adjust your position so you're working lower than elbow height. And on the opposite side, precision work may require you to work at heights above the elbow.

5. Reduce unnecessary motions.

Manual repetition can cause overuse injuries, so it's important to think about the motions you repeat throughout the day and find ways to reduce excessive motion. For example, rather than twisting your wrist to turn a screwdriver, is it possible to replace the screwdriver with a drill that will take the manual motion out of the task altogether? You can also look for opportunities to change your position or the layout of your work area to help you work more ergonomically.

6. Minimize fatigue caused by static load.

At your job, there may be tasks that require you to hold the same position for an extended period, which is known as static load. Static load can affect all parts of the body, such as the legs when standing for a long time or the shoulders when you need to hold your arms overhead for longer than a few seconds. These types of task can make your muscles tired and may eventually cause lasting discomfort even after the task is finished. Some ways you may be able to combat the fatigue caused by static load are to change the orientation of your work area, reposition your body, or even add extenders to your tools.

7. Minimize contact stress.

Contact stress occurs when a tool or surface routinely comes into contact with the same area of your body. Sometimes called pressure points, these areas of contact can cause discomfort. One example of contact stress is when you routinely squeeze a tool, like pliers, or hold a heavy item, like a nail gun, that puts pressure on an area of your hand. Adding padding, wearing gloves, or choosing tools with a cushioned grip can help. You may also consider adding anti-fatigue mats to standing surfaces to help alleviate contact stress on your heels.

8. Leave adequate clearance.

This principle is very simple—you need to have enough room for your head, knees, and feet. If you work in a seated position, adjust your seat to give yourself adequate legroom. Remove overhead obstructions to avoid bumping your head. Visibility also comes into play here. It's important that no matter where you're working or what equipment you're using, you have a clear view of what's going on around you.

9. Move and stretch throughout the day.

Staying in one position too long—whether sitting or standing—isn't healthy for the human body. Take breaks to exercise or stretch your muscles. If you sit for a long time, periodically find time to pause what you're doing and walk around. If you're on your feet all day, wear supportive footwear and use your breaks to rest. And if your job is physically demanding on certain parts of your body, it may help to stretch before jumping into strenuous tasks.

10. Keep your environment comfortable.

Work environments vary greatly depending on your industry and role, but some common items you may want to pay attention to are lighting, temperature, vibration, and noise. Look for ways to reduce glare or provide better lighting in low-light areas. Keep work areas at a comfortable temperature when possible, and when you're working outdoors, dress appropriately for the weather. And if tools create excessive noise or vibration, provide hearing protection and consider ways to dampen vibrating tools.

Aims of Ergonomics:

1. Health Benefits

People who work in ergonomic workplaces benefit from improved health. The effect of ergonomics starts within the cardiovascular system and spreads to other areas. Your heart will be healthier than it would be if you worked in a standard environment. Ergonomics can improve the health of your employees by reducing work-related injuries, most often caused by strains and over-exertion.

Ergonomic workstations can help you and your employees feel less tension in your body because you'll adjust the workstations to fit your height. A neutral position will prevent you from straining your eyes, neck, and back. Your legs can also benefit from better blood flow.

2. Improved Productivity

Ergonomic workplaces are efficient workplaces. Ergonomic workstations combine different ideas to improve workers' ability to complete their tasks—from organizing items and supplies to integrating computer equipment and monitors. An optimized workstation allows a worker to focus on their task and not be distracted by discomfort or a lack of organization. The more focused your employees are, the higher the level of productivity they can have.

3. Improved Mental Clarity

Reducing physical discomfort and improving your posture can improve your mental clarity and allow you to do your work more successfully. Ergonomics can also help you reduce stress and improve your concentration.

When you're feeling comfortable, you can focus better on your work. Ergonomics helps decrease pain, strengthen muscles, and increase blood flow. Combined, this can improve mental insight.

The improved moods and focus will allow you and your employees to be more productive and engaged in your work.

4. Decreased Pains

Ergonomics focuses on optimizing the design of the workplace, tools, and equipment to reduce strain on employees, minimize fatigue, and improve overall comfort and safety.

Ergonomics can also help improve posture and reduce the risk of musculoskeletal injuries, such as back pain, by providing ergonomically designed chairs, desks, other furniture, and adjustable workstations. By creating an ergonomically designed work environment, employers can help to ensure that employees remain healthy and productive.

5. Eliminates Hazards

Part of creating a more productive work environment is eliminating the daily hazards that can hurt your employees. Ergonomics contributes to identifying and eliminating hazards in the workplace by creating work environments that are tailored to fit the user.

Additionally, ergonomics helps to create a better environment by reducing distractions, providing suitable lighting and ventilation, and providing adjustable furniture and equipment, all of which help eliminate potential workplace hazards.

it is also a good idea to ask your employees about what hazards they see in their environment. By asking for their input, you're showing interest in them. Implementing the change will show them they've been heard, which will further help with employee engagement.

6. Quality Of Work Improves

The benefits of ergonomic workspaces range from employee well-being to the quality of work. Aches, pains, fatigue, and other problems can affect a worker. Ergonomics can eliminate those issues and help workers work.

Additionally, ergonomics can help ensure that employees are using the most effective tools and equipment to do their job and that they can reach and use the tools and equipment safely. A straightforward example is the way how proper lighting can reduce the number of mistakes that happen in a work process just by ensuring the worker can adequately see all details.

7. Reduce Absenteeism

Ergonomics can improve absenteeism by helping prevent workplace injuries that lead to missed workdays and creating a more comfortable working environment for employees. Ergonomic practices can also reduce employee fatigue and stress, which can be physical or psychological factors contributing to absenteeism.

Encourage your workers to take regular breaks, change postures frequently, and adjust their workstations to fit their body size and shape better.

Finally, promote positive health behaviors by providing resources and encouraging your employees to maintain a healthy diet and lifestyle.

8. Focus on Safety

Ergonomics will create a safer work environment and increase awareness. You'll remove hazards, improve workstations for less discomfort, and teach your employees to update their spaces with safety in mind.

Not to mention, the health benefits that come with ergonomics keep employees healthy at work. This will encourage safety on another level. You can keep your work consistent and stable by providing employees with a safe environment they can thrive in.

9. Increased Employee Satisfaction

The more you lean into the ergonomics culture, the more positive your work environment will be.

Ergonomics in the workplace can help improve employee satisfaction by reducing physical and mental stress. As a result, your employees will enjoy coming to work more than they did before, affecting those around them.

10. Lower Insurance Costs

Ergonomics in the workplace can help lower your insurance costs by reducing the risk of employees suffering from work-related injuries and illnesses. By reducing the number of Workers' Compensation claims, you could be able to save on insurance premiums.

Ergonomic improvements such as adjustable workstations, ergonomic chairs and keyboards, and improved lighting can help reduce employee fatigue and improve your overall working environment. In such an ergonomic work environment, your employees are less likely to become injured on the job.

In addition, implementing ergonomic policies and programs can provide you with greater legal protection in case of a worker injury.

➢ Types of Ergonomic Improvements

In general, ergonomic improvements are changes made to improve the fit between the demands of work tasks and the capabilities of your workers. There are usually many options for improving a particular manual handling task. It is up to you to make informed choices about which improvements will work best for particular tasks. There are two types of ergonomic improvements:

1. Engineering improvements
2. Administrative improvements

1. **Engineering Improvements:** These include rearranging, modifying, redesigning, providing or replacing tools, equipment, workstations, packaging, parts, processes, products, or materials.
2. **Administrative Improvements**: Observe how different workers perform the same tasks to get ideas for improving work practices or organizing the work. Then consider the following improvements:
   • Alternate heavy tasks with light tasks.
   • Provide variety in jobs to eliminate or reduce repetition (i.e., overuse of the same muscle groups).
   • Adjust work schedules, work pace, or work practices.
   • Provide recovery time (e.g., short rest breaks).
   • Modify work practices so that workers perform work within their power zone (i.e., above the knees, below the shoulders, and close to the body).
   • Rotate workers through jobs that use different muscles, body parts, or postures.

Administrative improvements, such as job rotation, can help reduce workers' exposures to risk factors by limiting the amount of time workers spend on "problem jobs." However, these measures may still expose workers to risk factors that can lead to injuries. For these reasons, the most effective way to eliminate "problem jobs" is to change them. This can be done by putting into place the appropriate engineering improvements and modifying work practices accordingly.

- **Risk Factors for bad ergonomics:**

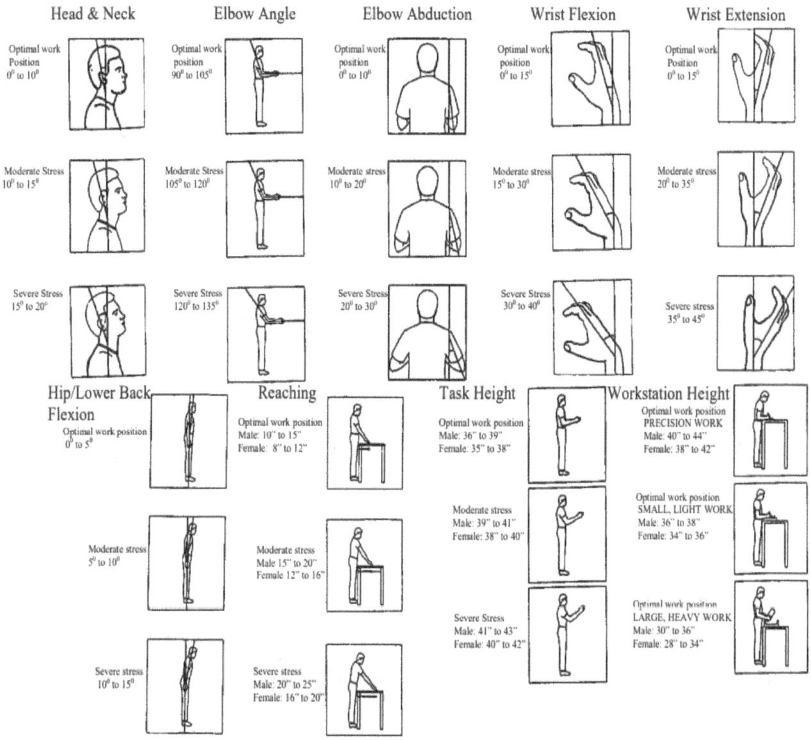

- **Ergonomic Assessment Checklist:**

*Note if there is a Yes checked in any block, please use page two to give a brief explanation of what the activity is or what the worker complaint was.

High Risk: If you answered Yes to #1 (and the shop has done nothing to fix it), if Yes to #2 or 3 and two other Yes's in #'s 4 through 15, or if Yes to six or more in #'s 4 through 15.
Medium Risk: If you answered Yes to #1 (and the shop has made changes), if Yes to #2 or 3 and one other Yes in #'s 4 through 15, or if Yes to three to five in #'s 4 through 15.
Low Risk: If no Yes's in #'s 1, 2, or 3 and less than 3 Yes's in #'s 4 through 15.

Ergonomic Assessment Checklist		
Risk Factors	**Yes**	**No**
1. Have any shop workers been previously diagnosed with any of the following CTD's: Carpal tunnel, Tendonitis, Tenosynovitis, De Quervain's disease, Trigger Finger, White finger, Hand Arm Segmental Vibration Syndrome, Muscle strains, or Back ailments?		
2. Have there been any worker complaints concerning ergonomic issues?		
3. Do employees perform high repetition tasks? (100 reps/hour to 2000 per/day)		
4. Do the employee's routine tasks require repeated heavy lifting? (>20 lbs) or occasional heavy lifting (>50 lbs)		
5. Are employees using awkwardly designed tools, which cause the worker to operate the tool outside of a neutral position for an extended period of time? (> 1 hour)		
6. Do employees perform tasks with an awkward head or neck position for an extended period of time? (1 to 3 hours)		
7. Do employees perform tasks that require awkward back angles to be held for extended periods of time (2 to 3 hours)? i.e...hunching, bending, or squatting		
8. Do employees perform tasks with an awkward elbow angle for an extended period of time (1 to 3 hours) or with extreme force application?		
9. Do employees perform tasks with an awkward elbow abduction angle for an extended period of time (1 to 3 hours) or with extreme force application?		
10. Do employees perform tasks with an awkward wrist flexion angle for an extended period of time (1 to 3 hours) or with extreme force application?		
11. Do employees perform tasks with an awkward wrist extension angle for an extended period of time (1 to 3 hours) or with extreme force application?		
12. Do employees perform tasks with an awkward back/hip flexion angle for an extended period of time (1 to 3 hours) or with extreme force application?		
13. Do employees perform tasks with an extreme reaching distance for an extended period of time (1 to 3 hours) or with extreme force application?		
14. Do employees perform tasks with an odd work station height (either standing or sitting) for an extended period of time (1-3 hours) or with extreme force application?		
15. Are high impact tools used routinely? i.e., riveters, bucking bars, or impact wrenches		
16. Are high vibration producing tools used routinely? i.e., die grinders, sanders, weed eaters		
17. Do employees perform tasks at an extreme height (high or low) for an extended period of time (1 to 3 hours) or with extreme force application?		
18. Are there any other areas of concern either from your observations or employee complaints?		

Ergonomic Survey Evaluation	Date	Activity Assessed

Ergonomic Survey Checklist Evaluation Explanation		
Question number & Activity Name	Brief Explanation – use this section if you answered yes to any questions on page 1 (please list corresponding question number) and briefly outline any risks associated with an activity	Risk Factors

Name of Assessor	Name of Reviewer

Computer Workstation Ergonomics:

Self-Assessment Checklist

The goal of this self-assessment is to help you set up your workstation for optimal comfort and performance. For more information, refer to the **National Institutes of Health, Office of Research Services, Division of Occupational Health and Safety website.**

Item	The Office Chair	Yes	No	N/A	Suggested Actions
1.	Can the height, seat and back of the chair be adjusted to achieve the posture outlined below?				• Obtain a fully adjustable chair
2.	Are your feet fully supported by the floor when you are seated?				• Lower the chair • Use a footrest
3.	Does your chair provide support for your lower back?				• Adjust chair back • Obtain proper chair • Obtain lumbar roll
4.	When your back is supported, you able to sit without feeling pressure from the chair seat on the back of your knees?				• Adjust seat pan • Add a back support
5.	Do your armrests allow you to get close to your workstation?				• Adjust armrests • Remove armrests
6.	Are your keyboard, mouse and work surface at your elbow height?				• Raise / lower workstation • Raise or lower keyboard • Raise or lower chair
7.	Are frequently used items within easy reach?				• Rearrange workstation
8.	Is the keyboard close to the front edge of the desk allowing space for the wrist to rest on the desk surface?				• Move keyboard to correct position
9.	When using your keyboard and mouse, are your wrists straight and your upper arms relaxed? *The keyboard should be flat and not propped up on keyboard legs as an angled keyboard may place the wrist in an awkward posture when keying.*				• Re-check chair, raise or lower as needed • Check posture • Check keyboard and mouse height
10.	Is your mouse at the same level and as close as possible to your keyboard?				• Move mouse closer to keyboard • Obtain larger keyboard tray if necessary
11.	Is the mouse comfortable to use?				• Rest your dominant hand by using the mouse with your non-dominant hand

12.	Is your monitor positioned directly in front of you?				• Reposition monitor
13.	Is your monitor positioned at least an arm's length away? Note: the monitor's location is dependent on the size of the monitor, the font, screen resolution and the individual user e.g. vision/use of bifocal spectacles etc.				• Reposition monitor • Seek an alternative monitor if necessary e.g. flat screen that uses less space
14.	Is your monitor height slightly below eye level?				• Add or remove monitor stand • Adjust monitor height
15.	Is your monitor and work surface free from glare?				• Windows at side of monitor • Adjust overhead lighting • Cover windows • Obtain antiglare screen
16.	Do you have appropriate light for reading or writing documents?				• Obtain desk lamp • Place on left if right-handed – place on right if left handed
17.	Are frequently used items located within the usual work area and items which are only used occasionally in the occasional work area?				• Rearrange worsktation

Item	Breaks	Yes	No	N/A	Suggested Actions
18.	Do you take postural breaks every 30 minutes? E.g. standing, walking to printer / fax etc.?				• Set reminders to take breaks
19.	Do you take regular eye breaks from looking at your monitor?				• Refocus on picture on wall every 30 minutes

Item	Accessories	Yes	No	N/A	Suggested Actions
20.	Is there a sloped desk surface or angle board for reading and writing tasks if required?				• Obtain an angle board
21.	Is there a document holder either beside the screen or between the screen and keyboard if required?				• Obtain document holder
22.	Are you using a headset or speakerphone if you are writing or keying while talking on the phone?				• Obtain a headset if using the phone and keyboard

Item	Laptop	Yes	No	N/A	Suggested Actions
23.	In the event of using a laptop computer for prolonged periods of time use of; • A full sized external keyboard and mouse; • Docking station with full sized monitor or a laptop stand				• Obtain appropriate laptop accessories

Item	"Hot Desking" (when applicable)	Yes	No	N/A	Suggested Actions
24.	Provided time, support and supervision to make above adjustments.				

Lifting and Material Handling

- What Manual Material Handling:

- According to the U.S. Department of Labor, handling is defi ned as: Seizing, holding, grasping, turning, or otherwise working with the hand or hands. Fingers are involved only to the extent that they are an extension of the hand, such as to turn a switch or to shift automobile gears.
- Lifting heavy items is one of the leading causes of injury in the workplace.
- In 2001, the Bureau of Labor Statistics reported that over 36 percent of injuries involving missed workdays were the result of shoulder and back injuries.
- Overexertion and cumulative trauma were the biggest factors in these injuries. Bending, followed by twisting and turning, were the more commonly cited movements that caused back injuries.
- Strains and sprains from lifting loads improperly or from carrying loads that are either too large or too heavy are common hazards associated with manually moving materials.
- When employees use smart lifting practices, they are less likely to suffer from back sprains, muscle pulls, wrist injuries, elbow injuries, spinal injuries and other injuries caused by lifting heavy objects.

Lifting Principles:

1. **Preparation** – Before lifting or carrying, plan out your lift.
   Think about:

- How heavy/awkward is the load? Should I use mechanical means (e.g. a hand truck) or another person to help me with this lift? Is it possible to break the load into smaller parts?
- Where am I going with the load? Is the path clear of obstructions, slippery areas, overhangs, stairs, and other uneven surfaces? Are there closed doors that need to be opened?

- Are there adequate handholds on the load? Do I need gloves or other personal protective equipment? Can I place the load in a container with better handholds? Should another person help me with the load?

Important Things to Remember.

- Use mechanical means (e.g. hand trucks, pushcarts, etc.) when possible for heavier or awkward loads. Remember to obtain training and authorization before using a forklift.
- It is easier and safer to push than to pull.
- Keep loads as close to the body as possible and do not twist while lifting, carrying or setting down a load. Nose, shoulders, hips and toes should all be facing the same direction.
- Minimize reaching.
- As a general rule, bend at the knees, not the hips.
- Get help when needed. Do not lift or carry things you don't feel comfortable with, no matter how light the load.
- Plan ahead for all parts of the lift: lifting, carrying and setting down.
- Try to utilize proper handholds while lifting. If an item does not have a good handhold, think of ways to remedy this, such as placing the item in a container with good handholds, creating a safe and proper handhold with an appropriate tool, etc.
- Use personal protective equipment where needed, such as gloves with good grip and steel-toed boots where appropriate.
- Implement rest breaks and job rotation for frequent and/or heavy lifting.
- Place items to be lifted within the "power zone". The power zone is close to the body, between the mid-thigh and mid-chest of the person doing the lifting. This is the area where the arms and back can lift the most with the least amount of effort.

Weight of Objects

- Heavier loads place greater stress on muscles, discs and vertebrae.
- Where possible, use mechanical means such as forklifts or hand trucks to transport heavy items.

- Ramps can be helpful in moving heavy items from one level to another. Materials that must be manually lifted should be placed at "power zone" height: about mid-thigh to mid-chest of the person doing the lifting.
- Ensure that proper lifting principles (see above) are used. Try to order supplies in smaller quantities and/or break loads up into smaller, lighter quantities where possible. Is the container itself heavy?
- Perhaps a smaller or lighter container is available.
- Limit weight you lift to no more than 50 pounds. When lifting loads heavier than 50 pounds, use two or more people to lift the load.

Awkward Postures

- Bending while lifting causes several problems for the back. It adds the weight of the upper body to the weight of the object being lifted. Bending and/or reaching moves the load away from the body and allows leverage to significantly increase the effective load on the back, leading to stress on the lower spine and muscle fatigue.
- Carrying loads on one shoulder, under an arm or in one hand creates uneven pressure on the spine.
- Move items close to the body and use the legs when lifting from a low location to minimize bending and reaching.
- Ensure proper housekeeping is taking place so that you may get as close to your lifting load as possible. Store and place materials that need to be manually lifted at the "power zone": mid-thigh to mid-chest height. This can be accomplished by placing objects on shelves, tables, racks or stacked pallets; or by using ladders or aerial lifts where necessary to elevate yourself and minimize overhead reaching.
- Roll-out decks in truck beds can be utilized to bring materials closer to the employee and eliminate the need to crawl into the back of a truck.
- Ensure that proper lifting principles (see above) are used, including avoiding twisting and holding the load close to the body.

High-Frequency and Long-Duration Lifting

- Holding items for long periods, even if loads are light, increases the risk of back and shoulder injury since muscles can be starved of nutrients and waste products can build up.
- Repeatedly exerting, such as when pulling wire, can fatigue muscles by limiting recuperation times. Inadequate rest periods do not allow the body time to recover.
- Plan ahead when beginning work that will require high-frequency and long-duration lifting. This way, the work can be organized in such a way so as to minimize the time workers spend holding loads.
- Adequate rest breaks can be planned in, as well as job rotation between employees. This includes both rotating tasks (employees trade off on differing tasks) and team work (two or more employees work together doing different parts of the same activity to reduce strain).
- Planning can also include the pre-assembly of work items to minimize the time spent handling them during the actual work.

Inadequate Handholds

- Inadequate handholds, such as boxes without handles or oddly-shaped loads, make lifting more difficult, move the load away from the body, lower lift heights and increase the risk of contact stress and of dropping the load.
- Where possible, utilize handholds such as handles, slots, or holes that provide enough room for gloved hands.
- Try to use materials that are packaged with proper handholds (your supplier may be able to provide different containers), or move materials into containers with good handholds.
- Wear protective equipment to avoid finger injuries and contact stress.
- Ensure that gloves fit properly and provide adequate grip.
- Suction devices are helpful in lifting junction boxes and other materials with smooth, flat surfaces. Other tools may be available that can create temporary handles.

Environmental Factors

- Be aware of extreme temperatures that can affect lifting and material handling. For example, muscle flexibility decreases in cold temperatures, and hot temperatures can lead to heat stress. Low visibility or poor lighting increases the chance of trips and falls.
- Do what you can to adjust work schedules to minimize exposure to extreme temperatures or low visibility.
- Wear appropriate clothing for the temperature in which you will be working. Drink lots of water to avoid dehydration in excessive heat.
- Provide proper lighting for areas with low light and try to perform work during daylight hours when possible.

2. **LIFTING:**

- Get as close to the load as possible.
- Try to keep your elbows and arms close to your body.
- Keep your back straight during the lift by tightening the stomach muscles, bending at the knees, keeping the load close and centered in front of you, and looking up and ahead.
- Get a good handhold and do not twist while lifting. Do not jerk; use a smooth motion while lifting. If the load is too heavy to allow this, find someone to help you with the lift.

3. **CARRYING:**

    - Do not twist or turn the body; instead, move your feet to turn.
    - Your hips, shoulders, toes and knees should stay facing the same direction.
    - Keep the load as close to your body as possible with your elbows close to your sides.
    - If you feel fatigued, set the load down and rest for a few minutes.
    - Don't let yourself get so fatigued that you cannot perform proper setting down and lifting technique for your rest.

4. **Setting Down.**

- Set the load down in the same way you picked it up, but in the reverse order.
- Bend at the knees, not the hips.
- Keep your head up, your stomach muscles tight, and do not twist your body. Keep the load as close to the body as possible.
- Wait until the load is secure to release your handhold.

Avoid lifting from the floor whenever possible. If you must lift from the floor, do not bend at the waist. The techniques shown below help the worker to keep the spine in a safer position while lifting from the floor.

Caution: This technique may be effective only if loads are small, light weight, and can easily fit between the knees.

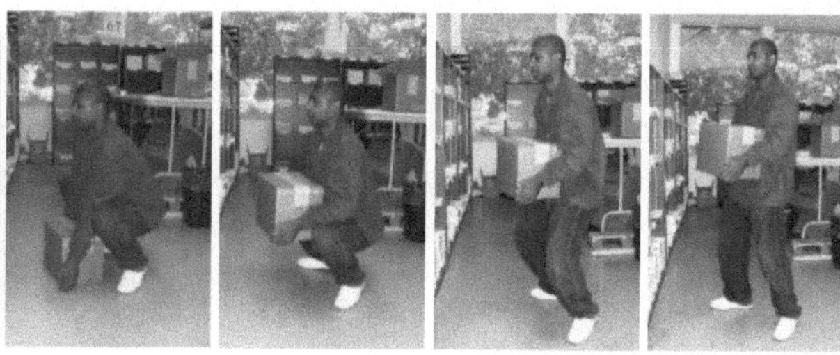

Keep the load close to your body and lift by pushing up with your legs.

Use team lifting as a temporary measure until a more permanent improvement can be found. If possible, try to find a co-worker of similar height to help with the lift.

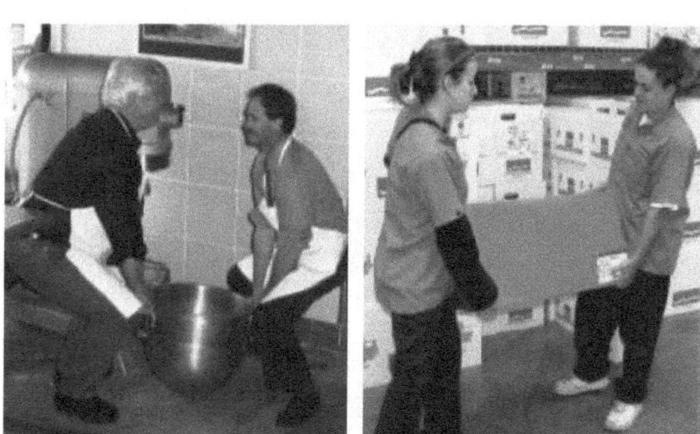

Team lifting can reduce the load in half. Discuss your lifting plan so you don't make surprise movements.

Use a turntable. Rotate the turntable to bring the container closer. Always work from the side closest to the load.

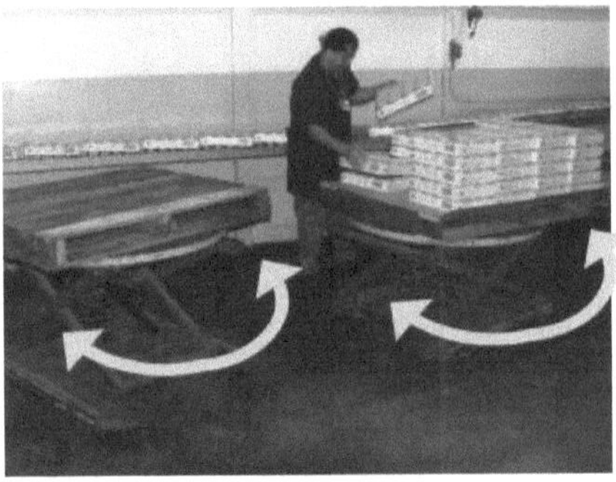

Turntable on a load leveler

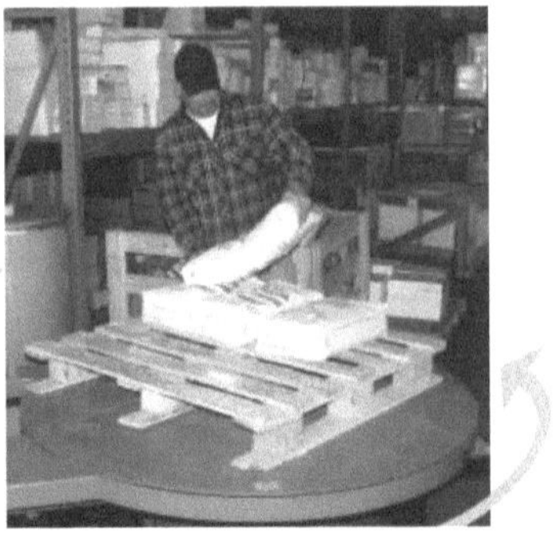

A fixed-height turntable for pallets with short low stacks.

Raise the worker so that the container is grasped 30"– 40" from the surface the worker is standing on.

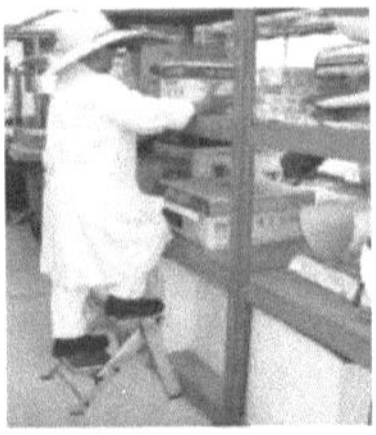

Use a step stool.

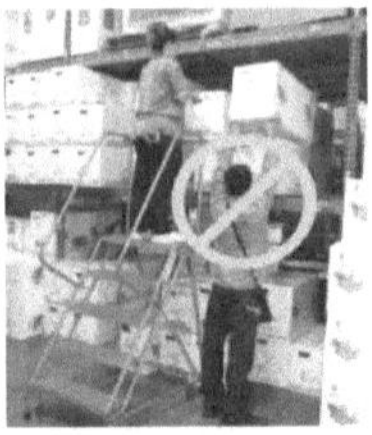

Use portable steps.

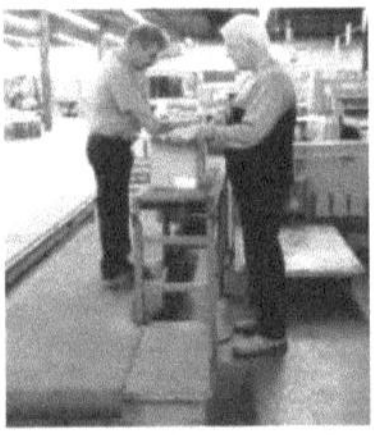

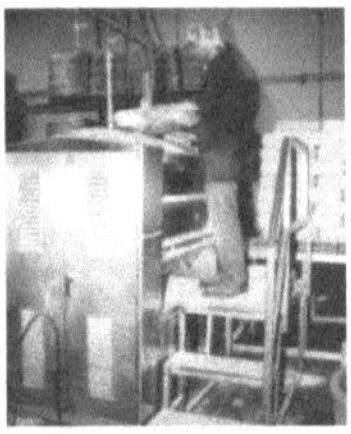

Use catwalks or platforms.

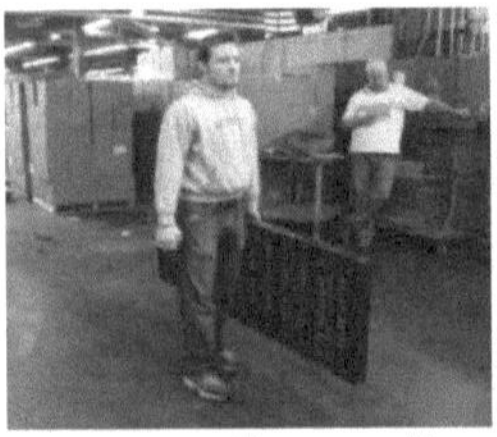

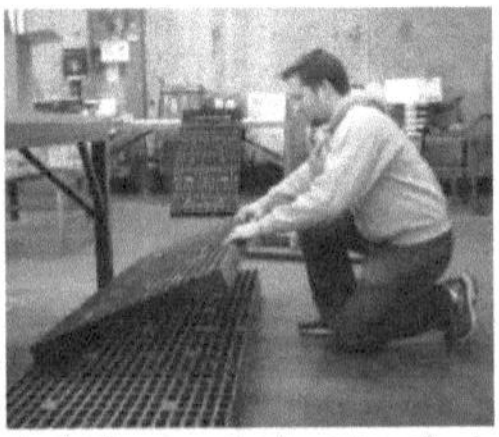

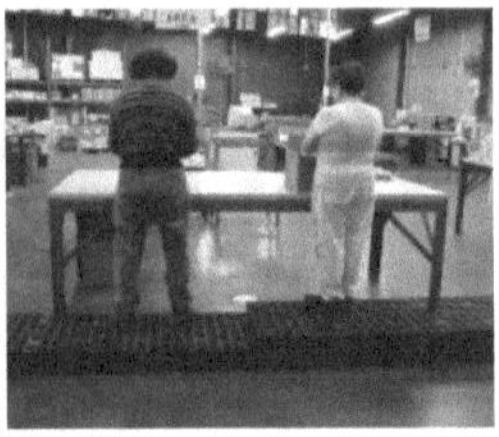

Use a portable work platform and adjust it to the height of the worker.

> ! *Caution:* When using portable steps, stools, catwalks, or other work platforms, follow all manufacturers' recommendations for proper use. Use only equipment appropriate to the weight, size, and shape of the load being handled.

Support the container on or against a fixed object, rack, or stand while pouring the contents.

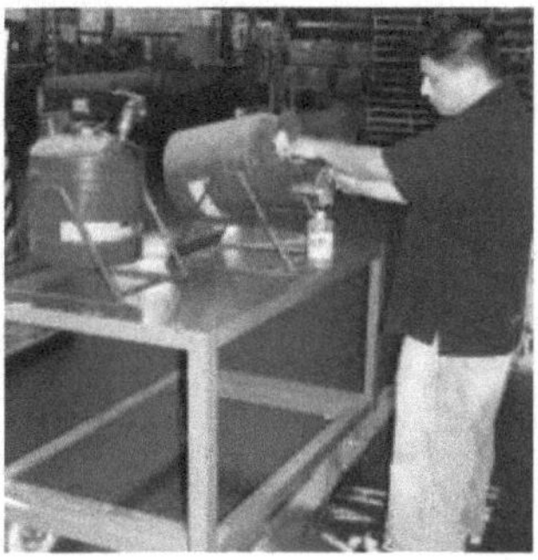

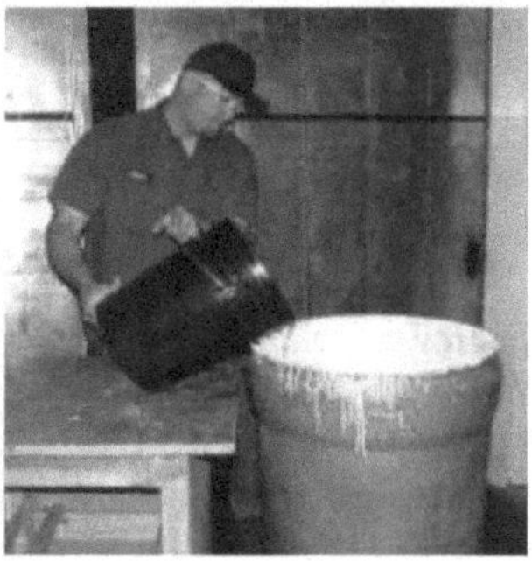

Use a removable plate or a work surface to support the container while pouring the contents into the receptacle.

Instead of lifting and pouring from the drum, insert a siphon or a pump.

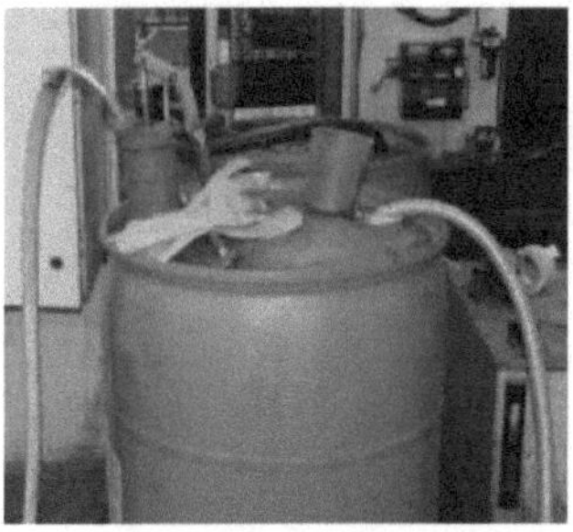

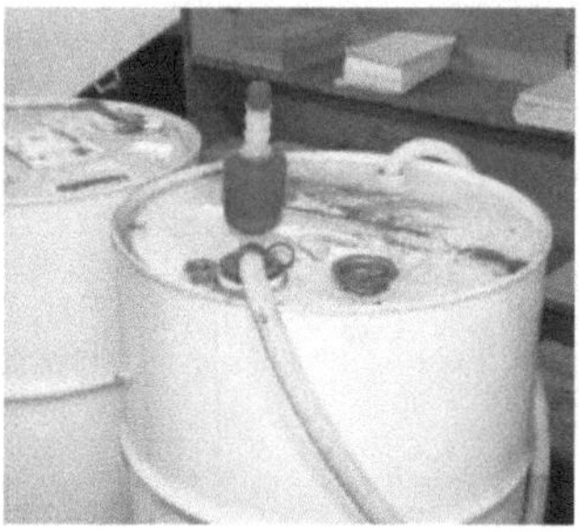

! *Caution:* To prevent cross-contamination, chemical incompatibility, and flammability hazards, do not interchange pumps or siphons among different containers.

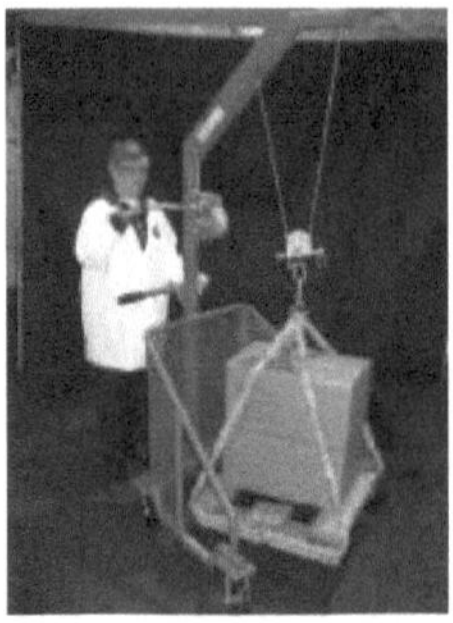

A portable hoist or "cherry picker" is manually operated. It is convenient for occasional spot-lifting of heavy loads.

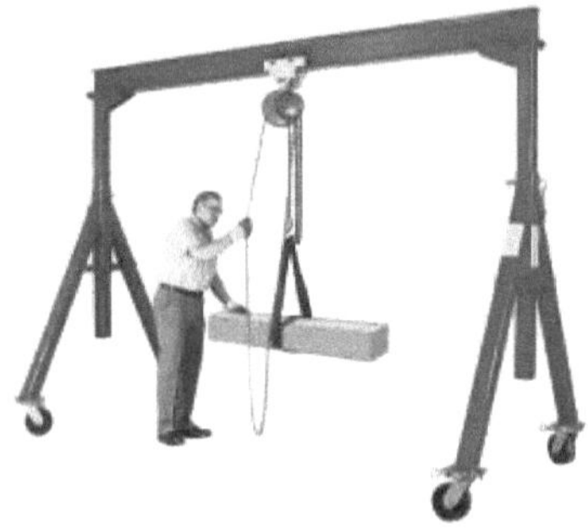

Portable gantry cranes are adjustable in height. They can be fitted with manual, electric, or pneumatic hoists for moving heavy loads over short distances.

NIOSH Manual Material Handling (MMH) Checklist:

This checklist is not designed to be a comprehensive risk assessment technique but rather as a tool to quickly identify potential problem jobs. Additional risk factors may exist that are not accounted for in this checklist. It is common practice to follow up checklist observations with more precise techniques to confirm problem risk factors.

"No" responses indicate potential problem areas that should be investigated further.

1. Are the weights of loads to be lifted judged acceptable by the workforce?	yes	no
2. Are materials moved over minimum distances?	yes	no
3. Is the distance between the object load and the body minimized?	yes	no
4. Are walking surfaces level?	yes	no
wide enough?	yes	no
clean and dry?	yes	no
5. Are objects easy to grasp?	yes	no
stable?	yes	no
able to be held without slipping?	yes	no
6. Are there handholds on these objects?	yes	no
7. When required, do gloves fit properly?	yes	no
8. Is the proper footwear worn?	yes	no
9. Is there enough room to maneuver?	yes	no
10. Are mechanical aids used whenever possible?	yes	no
11. Are working surfaces adjustable to the best handling heights?	yes	no
12. Does material handling avoid:	yes	no
movements below knuckle height and above shoulder height?	yes	no
static muscle loading?	yes	no
sudden movements during handling?	yes	no
twisting at the waist?	yes	no
extended reaching?	yes	no
13. Is help available for heavy or awkward lifts?	yes	no
14. Are high rates of repetition avoided by job rotation?	yes	no
self-pacing?	yes	no
sufficient pauses?	yes	no
15. Are pushing or pulling forces reduced or eliminated?	yes	no
16. Does the employee have an unobstructed view of handling the task?	yes	no
17. Is there a preventive maintenance program for equipment?	yes	no
18. Are workers trained in correct handling and lifting procedures?	yes	no

Ergonomics Checklist — Material Handling

The checklist presented below is from the book Kodak's Ergonomic Design for People at Work (adapted from material developed by the Chemical Manufacturers Association). It helps users to identify any job risk factors that may be present in the job. This checklist is applicable to jobs requiring the routine handling of objects of 10 pounds or more.

Job/Task: ---------------------------- Dept: -----------------------------------

Date: ------------------------------- Analyst: ---------------------------------

Before ------------------------------- After: ---------------------------------

Directions: Review each condition for the job/task of interest and for each condition that frequently occurs, place an X in the "Concern" column as appropriate. Add comments as appropriate.

Condition	X if a Concern	Comments
REPETITION		
High-speed process line or work presentation rates		
Similar motions every few seconds		
Observed signs of fatigue		
WORKSTATION DESIGN		
Work surface too high or low		
Location of materials promotes reaching		
Angle/orientation of containers promotes non-neutral positions		
Spacing between adjacent transfer surfaces promotes twisting		
Obstructions prevent direct access to load/unload points		
Obstacles on floor prevent a clear path of travel		
Floor surfaces are uneven, slippery, or sloping		
Hoists or other power lifting devices are needed but not available		

Condition	X if a Concern	Comments
LIFTING AND LOWERING		
Heavy objects need to be handled		
Handling bulky or difficult-to-grasp objects		
Handling above the shoulders or below the knees		
Lifting to the side or unbalanced lifting		
Placing objects accurately/precisely		
Sudden, jerky movements during handling		
One-handed lifting		
Long-duration exertions (static work)		
PUSHING/PULLING/CARRYING		
Forceful pushing/pulling of carts or equipment required		
Brakes for stopping hand carts/handling aids are needed but not available		
Carts or equipment design promotes non-neutral postures		
Long-distance carrying (carts not available)		
CONTAINERS/MATERIALS		
Lack adequate handles or gripping surfaces		
Are unbalanced, unstable, or contents shift		
Obstructs leg movement when being carried		
OTHER		
Inappropriate work techniques used		
Buildup of process material /product increases worker effort		
Personal protective equipment needed but not available/used		
TOTAL SCORE (Optional)		*To score, add up the total number of Xs identified.*

The Revised NIOSH Lifting Equation (RNLE):

The Revised Lifting Equation (RNLE) is a tool to calculate risk for work-related musculoskeletal disorders (WMSDs). The equation can be used to calculate both single and multiple manual lifting tasks. Using the equation can reduce the incidence of low back injuries in workers.

NIOSH created the RNLE because many workers are responsible for manually lifting and moving objects on the job. These workers are in numerous occupations and industries. Exposure to repetitive lifting puts workers at risk for developing WMSDs. Understanding how much workers can safely lift is important to preventing those injuries.

Key benefits of using the RNLE

The RNLE helps employers make informed decisions about mitigating potential hazards to their workers' musculoskeletal health. The RNLE benefits employers and safety professionals by:

- Providing guidelines for designing safe lifting tasks
- Serving as a risk assessment tool
- Helping raise workers' awareness about their job tasks
- Collecting quantitative lifting data for research

NIOSH Lifting Equation:

RWL = LC (51) x HM x VM x DM x AM x FM x CM

where LC is the load constant (23 kg) and other factors in the equation are:

- HM, the Horizontal Multiplier factor
- VM, the Vertical Multiplier factor
- DM, the Distance Multiplier factor
- FM, the Frequency Multiplier factor
- AM, the Asymmetric Multiplier factor
- CM, the Coupling Multiplier factor
- RWL, the Recommended Weight Limit

Recommended Weight Limit (RWL): "Is this weight too heavy for the task?"
The primary product of the NIOSH equation is the Recommended Weight Limit (RWL), which defines the maximum acceptable weight (load) that nearly all healthy employees could lift over the course of an 8-hour shift without increasing the risk of musculoskeletal disorders (MSD) to the lower back.

Lifting Index (LI): "How significant is the risk?"
In addition, a Lifting Index (LI) is calculated to provide a relative estimate of the level of physical stress and MSD risk associated with the manual lifting tasks evaluated. A Lifting Index value of 1.0 or less indicates a nominal risk to healthy employees. A Lifting Index greater than 1.0 denotes that the task is high risk for some fraction of the population. As the LI increases, the level of injury risk increases correspondingly. Therefore, the goal is to design all lifting jobs to accomplish an LI of 1.0 or less.

Uses of RWL and LI: The RWL and LI can be used to guide or engineer lifting task design in the following ways:

- Individual multipliers that determine the RWL can be used to identify specific weaknesses in the design.
- The LI can be used to estimate the relative physical stress and injury risk for a task or job. The higher the LI value, the smaller the percentage of workers capable of safely performing these lifting job demands. So using the LI, injury risk of two or more job designs could be compared.
- The LI can also be used to prioritize ergonomic redesign efforts.
- For example, jobs can be ranked by LI and a control strategy can be implemented based on a priority order of the jobs or individual lifting tasks.
-

The following task variables are evaluated to calculate the multipliers that are used in the NIOSH equation to determine the RWL. Here are some quick explanations and guidelines that you can use to gather the needed measurements:
Horizontal Location of the Hands (H) – Measure and record the horizontal location of the hands at both the start (origin) and end (destination) of the lifting task. Measure and record the horizontal location of the hands at the end (destination) of the lifting task only if significant control is required. The horizontal location is determined by measuring the

distance between the point projected on the floor directly below the mid-point of the hands grasping the object (load center), and the mid-point of a line between the inside ankle bones as pictured below:

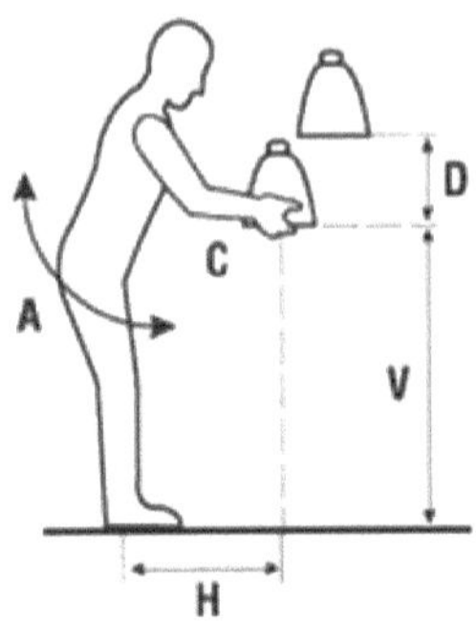

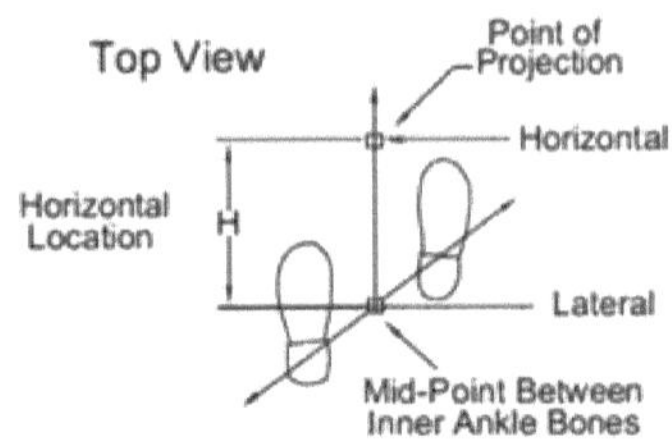

Vertical Location of the Hands (V) – Measure and record the vertical location of the hands above the floor at the start (origin) and end (destination) of the lifting task. The vertical location is measured from the floor (or standing surface) to the vertical mid-point between the hand grasps as defined by large middle knuckle (3rd MCP joint) of the hand.

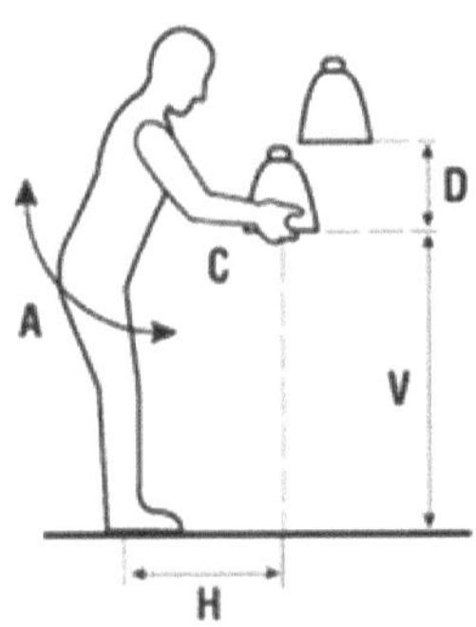

Vertical Travel Distance (D) – The vertical travel distance of a lift is determined by subtracting the vertical location (V) at the start of the lift from the vertical location (V) at the end of the lift. For a lowering task, subtract the V location at the end from the V location at the start. If you're using ErgoPlus Industrial, there's no need to worry about this one, the calculator will do this work for you.

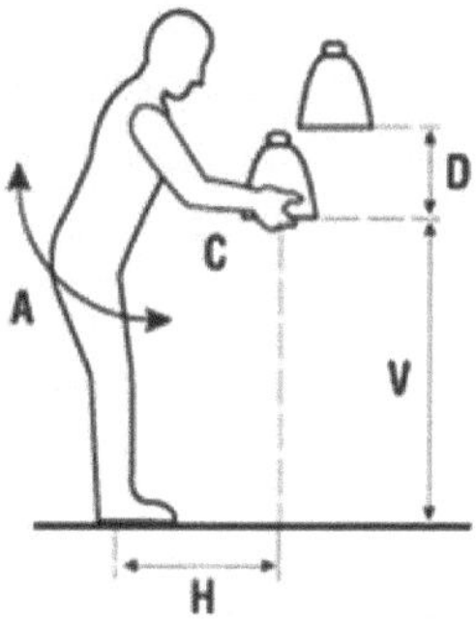

Asymmetric Angle (A) – Measure the degree to which the body is required to twist or turn during the lifting task. The asymmetric angle is the amount (in degrees) of trunk and shoulder rotation required by the lifting task. Note: Sometimes the twisting is not caused by the physical aspects of the job design, but rather by the employee using poor body mechanics. If this is the case, no twisting (0 degrees) is required by the job. If twisting is required by the design of the job, determine the number of degrees the back and body trunk must twist or rotate to accomplish the lift. (i.e. 90° as pictured below)

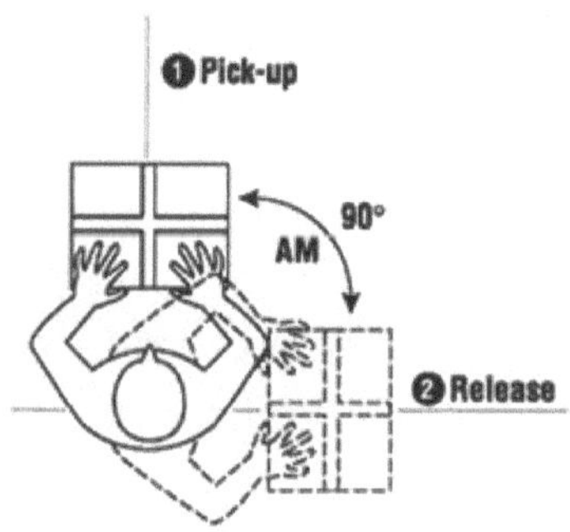

Coupling (C) – Determine the classification of the quality of the coupling between the worker's hands and the object as good, fair, or poor (1, 2, or 3). A good coupling will reduce the maximum grasp forces required and increase the acceptable weight for lifting, while a poor coupling will generally require higher maximum grasp forces and decrease the acceptable weight for lifting.

- 1 = Good – Optimal design containers with handles of optimal design, or irregular objects where the hand can be easily wrapped around the object.
- 2 = Fair – Optimal design containers with handles of less than optimal design, optimal design containers with no handles or cut-outs, or irregular objects where the hand can be flexed about 90°.
- 3 = Poor – Less than optimal design container with no handles or cut-outs, or irregular objects that are hard to handle and/or bulky (e.g. bags that sag in the middle).

Frequency (F) – Determine the average number of lifts per minute of the lifting task being evaluated, this is the lifting frequency. This information can often be verified by asking for average production rates from a group leader, supervisor, or production manager. You can also accomplish this by determining the number of lifts per minute during a short sampling period. NIOSH recommends a 15-minute sampling or observation period. The Frequency (F) value will be between 0.2 lifts/minute and 15 lifts/minute. For lifting tasks with a frequency less than .2 lifts per minute (>1 lift every 5 minutes), you will use the minimum frequency of .2 lifts/minute.

Load (L) – Determine the weight of the object lifted. If necessary, use a scale to determine the exact weight. If the weight of the load varies from lift to lift, you should record the average and maximum weights lifted.

Duration (Dur) – Determine the lifting duration as classified into one of three categories: Enter 1 for short-duration, 2 for moderate-duration and 8 for long-duration as follows:

- 1 = Short – lifting ≤ 1 hour with recovery time ≥ 1.2 X work time
- 2 = Moderate – lifting between 1 and 2 hours with recovery time ≥ 0.3 X lifting time
- 8 = Long – lifting between 2 and 8 hours with standard industrial rest allowances

Office Ergonomics

- Many jobs require a 40-hour work week, which, taken over a long enough period of time constitutes a significant portion of a worker's life.
- Poor ergonomics can result in overstraining the body over time, causing discomfort or injury, potentially for life. Injuries like carpal tunnel syndrome can be caused by poor posture and lead to potentially irreversible nerve damage in the arm or wrist.
- Ergonomics can help prevent injuries by providing tools to reduce strain and keep the body in a healthier posture.
- Proper ergonomics is important in the workplaces of any industry. In addition to reducing the risk of injury, ergonomics positively impacts productivity and job satisfaction.
- Employees are more likely to be engaged with their work and perform at a higher calibre when they feel comfortable and supported in their workspace. These benefits reach beyond industrial workspaces and prevention of bodily injury.
- Ergonomic workstations in office settings can also help reduce eye strain, headaches, and other common workplace discomforts, improving employee satisfaction, performance, and productivity.
- Musculoskeletal disorders (MSDs) are injuries that affect the body's muscles, tendons, and nerves.
- These injuries are often caused by overexertion, awkward postures, and repetitive motions. They can result in pain, discomfort, and long-term disability, which can be costly for the employee and the employer.
- Employers can reduce the risk of MSDs and other workplace injuries by creating an ergonomically sound workspace.
- One extremely common example of an MSD is carpal tunnel syndrome, a condition where nerves become compressed at the wrist. This compression often results in pain or tingling in the hand and arm. Repetitive hand movements, such as typing, often cause carpal tunnel, and the damage can be exacerbated by poor ergonomics in the workplace. For example, if a worker's keyboard or mouse is not at the correct angle or height, it can cause strain on the wrists and hands over time.
- Poor posture can cause headaches, neck pain, shoulder pain, and stiffness. For example, if a desk or chair is at the wrong height, it can cause the employee to hunch

over, leading to poor posture and pain over time. Poor placement of a computer monitor or inadequate lighting can cause eye strain, headaches, and even vision problems.

- Alongside physical consequences for workers, ignoring workplace ergonomics safety can also have negative consequences for employers. Discomfort and pain caused by poor ergonomics can reduce productivity and increase absenteeism. For example, employees who experience discomfort or pain may need to take more frequent breaks, work more slowly, or take time off to recover from an injury caused by workplace strain.
- Workplace injuries and conditions caused by poor ergonomics can increase healthcare costs for both employees and employers. For example, MSDs and repetitive strain injuries sometimes require medical treatment, physical therapy, or surgery, which can add to a company's healthcare and workers' compensation costs. Employees who take time off or leave their workplaces due to injuries can incur lost wages and other costs.

➢ **Office Ergonomics Checklist**

Creating an ergonomically sound workspace is essential for promoting the health and safety of employees who work in an office setting. The following office ergonomics checklist provides a guide for optimizing safety and comfort, reducing the risk of workplace injuries, and promoting productivity and job satisfaction in office workspaces.

- **Chair Height** – Improper chair height can cause discomfort and pain in the hips, legs, and lower back. To achieve a proper sitting posture, individuals should raise their chair high to allow the feet to rest flat on the floor, thighs to be parallel to the floor, and hips to be level with the knees.
- **Desk Height** – To avoid wrist strain, which can lead to carpal tunnel syndrome, users should maintain desks at a height that allows them to keep their forearms parallel to the floor and their wrists in a neutral position. In the event the desk is too high, the user should utilize a footrest to adjust the seating position. If multiple individuals with different heights share a desk or workstation, a height-adjustable desk could be an ergonomic solution.
- **Monitor Placement** – Position the computer monitor so the top of the screen is at or slightly below eye level, which will help reduce neck and eye strain.

- **Keyboard and Mouse Placement** – Place the keyboard and mouse in a position that allows elbows to be at a 90-degree angle and wrists to be straight. Avoid placing these items too far away, which can cause overreaching and shoulder strain.
- **Lighting** – Use adjustable lighting to reduce glare and prevent eye strain and discomfort. Avoid positioning a screen in front of a bright light source.
- **Ambient Noise Reduction** – Ambient noise can be distracting and cause stress in the workplace. Consider using noise-cancelling headphones or white noise machines to reduce distractions.

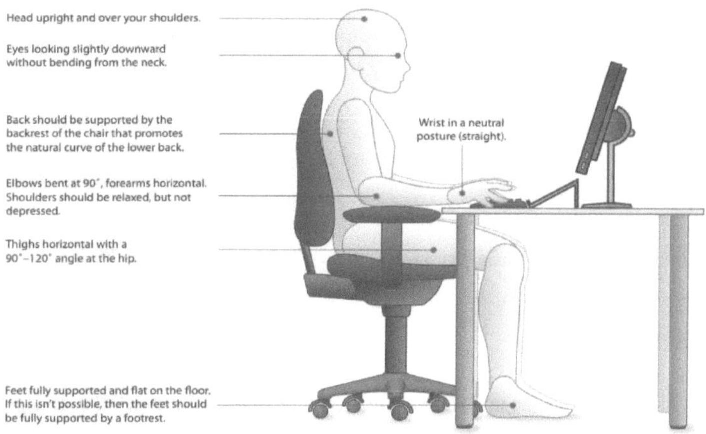

Office Ergonomics Equipment

- In today's workplace, ergonomic equipment is becoming increasingly comAccording to a 2020 study in *Applied Ergonomics,* such equipment has been proven to reduce the risk of work-related injuries from job hazards and increase employee satisfaction and productivity. When selecting ergonomic equipment for a workplace, it's important to ensure employees receive training on properly adjusting and using the equipment to maximize its benefits.
- While office ergonomic equipment may seem like a luxury expense, it should be considered not only as a means of reducing costs from losses of productivity or workplace injuries, but also as a means to improve employee morale and productivity.
- Posture is the most important aspect when looking at workstation design.

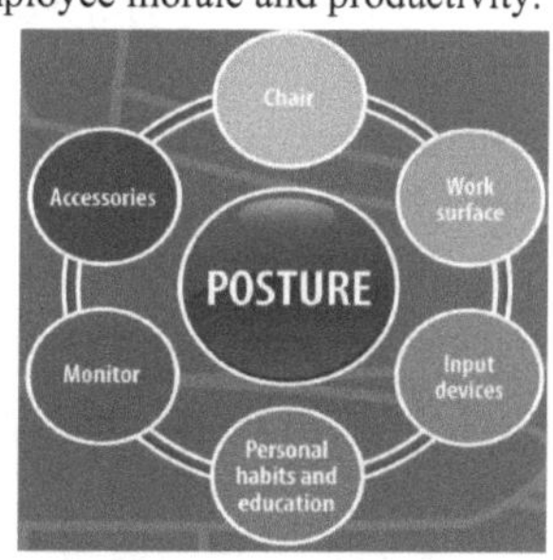

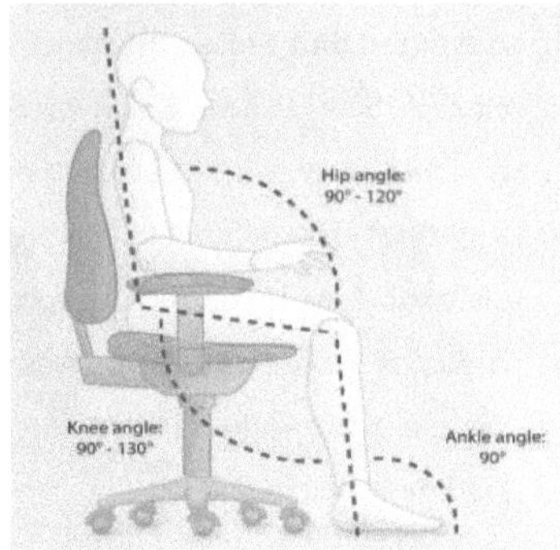

- Chairs, work surfaces, input devices, personal habits and education, monitors and accessories can help or hinder in maintaining optimal posture, but they cannot cause optimal posture.

For example, having an adjustable chair does not guarantee, but merely facilitates, optimal posture. It is up to the user to identify their optimal posture, and how to make workstation adjustments to help maintain it.

➢ **CHAIRS:**

- When workstations cause discomfort, the first-place people typically look is their chair. There are some basic guidelines to look for in a well-fitted office chair.
- **ARMRESTS:**

Armrests should be adjusted to elbow height. Too high, the shoulders will be shrugged; too low, the shoulders will be depressed. However, the armrests should not prevent the chair from being positioned close to the desk, nor restrict natural movements. If your armrests cannot be adjusted to allow for this, then consider removing or replacing them. Also, keep in mind that soft armrests will minimize contact stresses on your elbows. Gel wraps can be purchased to go over armrests that may be too hard.

- **BACK SUPPORT**

When sitting, adjust the height of the backrest so the lumbar pad supports the natural curve of your lower back (lumbar curve). The tilt of the back support should allow you to sit with your upper body slightly reclined.

- **DEPTH**

When sitting, the seat pan (part of the chair you sit on) should allow you to use the back support without the front of the seat pressing against the back of your knees. If the seat is too deep, try a back support or lumbar roll to reduce the size of the seat pan. Some chairs have adjustable seat pans.

- **HEIGHT**

While standing, adjust the height of the chair so the highest point of the seat is just below your kneecap. This should allow your feet to rest firmly on the floor when seated. If you feel pressure near the back of the seat, raise your chair. If you feel pressure near the front of the seat, lower your chair. The goal is to evenly distribute your weight.

- **SEAT TILT**

Seat tilt can be adjusted to improve your comfort. This will also affect your weight distribution.

- **WIDTH**

The seat pan should be wide enough so it does not apply pressure to your thighs, but narrow enough to be able to reach the armrests when they are properly adjusted.

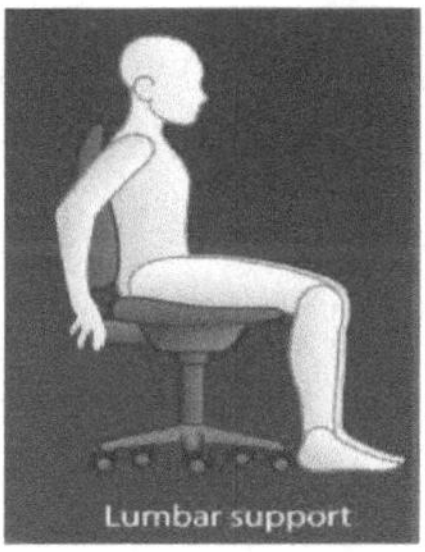

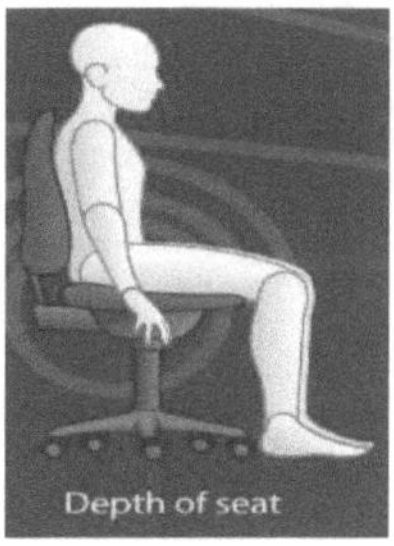

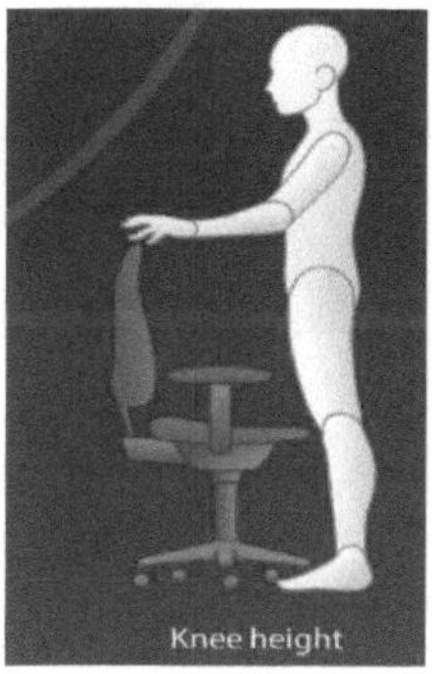

- **WORK SURFACE:**

Like your chair, your work surface should fit you. Once you have adjusted your chair, you can determine the appropriate height for your work surface. The top of your work surface should be at your elbow height. Make any necessary adjustments by raising or lowering your work surface. If your work surface cannot be raised or lowered to accommodate your elbow height, you can raise your chair and use a footrest. The footrest should be large enough for both feet. Please note that a footrest can restrict movement and make it more difficult for a user to adjust chair features. If necessary, a keyboard tray can be used to bring the keyboard and mouse to elbow height. A keyboard tray should be stable, height adjustable, have room for both the keyboard and mouse on the same surface, and should not limit legroom. Items used frequently should be located within easy reach. Keeping infrequently used items out of reach will encourage you to get out of your chair for them - this will promote blood circulation and reduce overall discomfort.

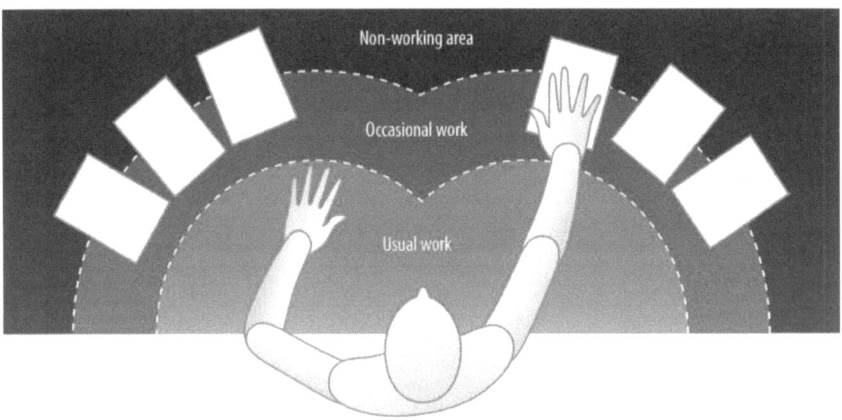

- **INPUT DEVICES:**

There are several different types of input devices. The most popular and widely -used are the keyboard and mouse.

When using a keyboard and mouse, your upper arms should be relaxed and by your sides, your elbows bent at a right angle (90 degrees) and your wrists straight.

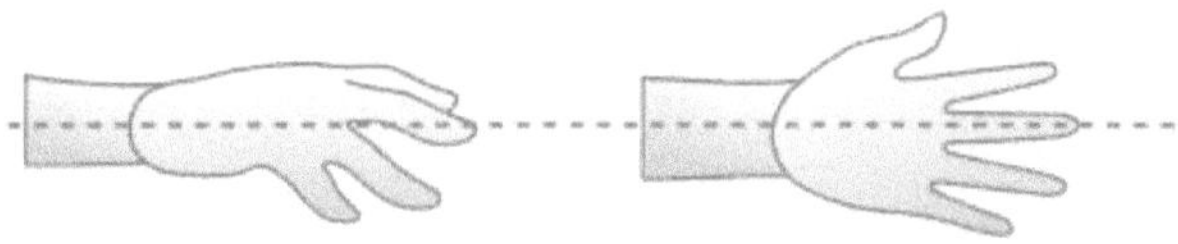

Neutral wrist posture

- **KEYBOARD**

There are many types of keyboards designed to place the hands in a more neutral position to help prevent injuries. The effectiveness of alternative keyboards depends on the user and the type of work being performed.

- **MOUSE**

The mouse should be at the same surface/height as the keyboard and easy to reach. Users are encouraged to alternate mouse usage between the left and right hands (by changing hands you are using different muscles, thereby reducing the risk of injury). Users can go to the operating system control panel to adjust the button assignment so the primary button is the one closest to the keyboard.

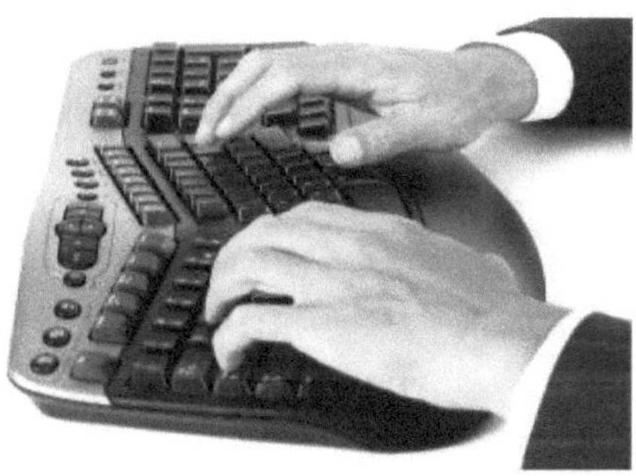

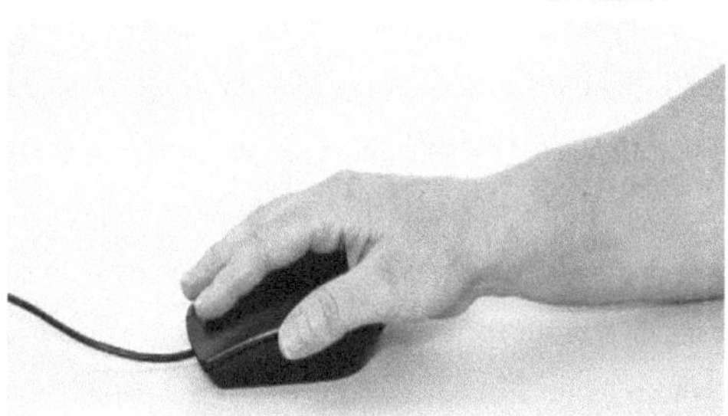

- **MONITOR:**

    - **DISTANCE**

How far you sit from your monitor will depend on your vision and the size and resolution of your monitor. As a general rule, it is best to move the monitor as far away as possible and increase the font size. The CSA Standard on office ergonomics specifies that the distance should be between 50-100 cm.

    - **HEIGHT AND LOCATION**

The monitor should be positioned directly in front of you with the top of the monitor just below eye level. A common practice is to place the monitor on a computer case or stand (sometimes even stacks of paper and phonebooks); however, this places the monitor too high for most individuals and causes neck discomfort and pain. The monitor should also be tilted 10-15 degrees for proper accommodation of the normal line of sight.

    - **CORRECTIVE LENSES**

If you wear progressive lenses, the monitor may need to be even lower to maintain optimal posture. Depending on vision levels, and the amount and type of computer work being done, corrective lenses specifically for computer use may be considered. Your optometrist will be able to determine the best solution, based on your needs.

    - **LIGHTING AND GLARE**

The CSA standard on office ergonomics specifies light levels between 75-300 lux for computer-based tasks. Higher light levels may cause glare on work surfaces and monitors. To test for glare, turn off your monitor – if the screen provides reflections, you have glare. Since this glare is caused by light shining directly onto your screen, check its source. If it is a window, this can be corrected by positioning your monitor so that your line of sight is parallel to the window. If this is not practical, cover the window with blinds. If lighting is causing the glare, the lights should be shaded or removed. A desk lamp will provide the extra lighting to see paper documents, while avoiding excessive light near the monitor. If you are right-handed, the lamp should be on the left side (and vice versa) to reduce shadows. Take regular eye breaks. Get into the habit of taking your eyes off the screen every few minutes and focusing on something far away. You can also move your eyes up and down, and side-to-side without moving your head. This will help decrease eye strain. For more information on lighting, refer to the Canadian Centre for Occupational Health and Safety website.

- **DUAL MONITORS**

When using two monitors, your screens should be positioned side-by side, at the same height and with a slight "V" angle. You should be positioned at the centre of your "screen real estate." This is the spot at the middle of the full width of your two screens

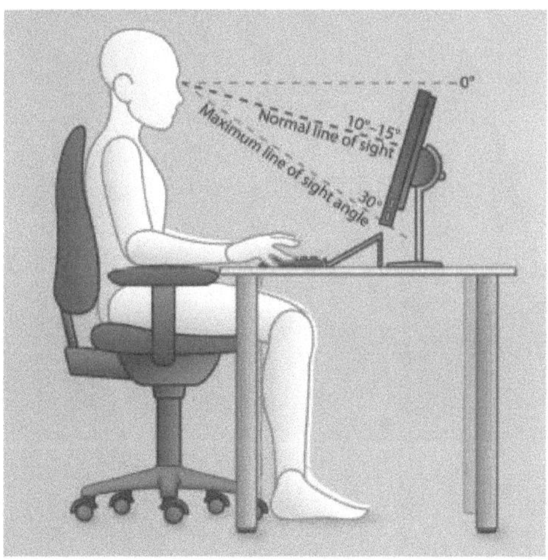

OTHER ACCESSORIES

- **PALM REST / SUPPORT**

Palm rests are designed to raise the palms and keep the wrists in a neutral position. They are not meant to be positioned under the wrists; this will cause pressure on the underside of the wrists which will compress the tissues and blood vessels, resulting in decreased blood flow and increased injury risk.

- **DOCUMENT HOLDER**

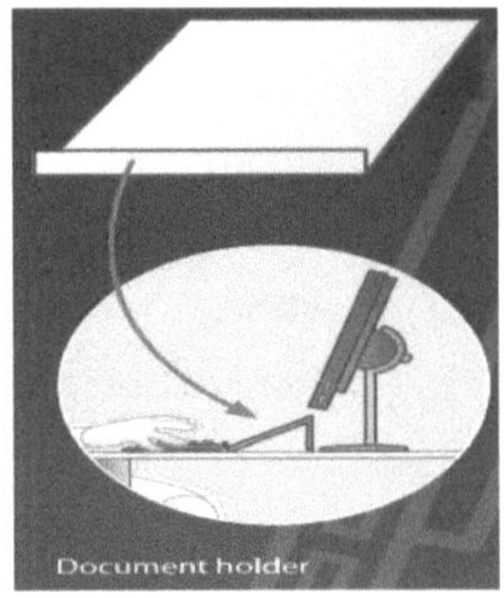

When frequent data entry from a source document is required, provide a sloped document holder positioned directly in front of the user to promote optimal posture while viewing the document.

- **PHONE**

Keep your phone within easy reach. If you use it while typing or writing, use a headset or a speakerphone to avoid awkward positioning of your neck.

- **STRETCHES:**

Sitting at a computer for long periods often causes neck and shoulder stiffness and, occasionally, lower back pain. Do these stretches every hour or so throughout the day, or whenever you feel stiff. Be sure to move around frequently – you'll feel better!

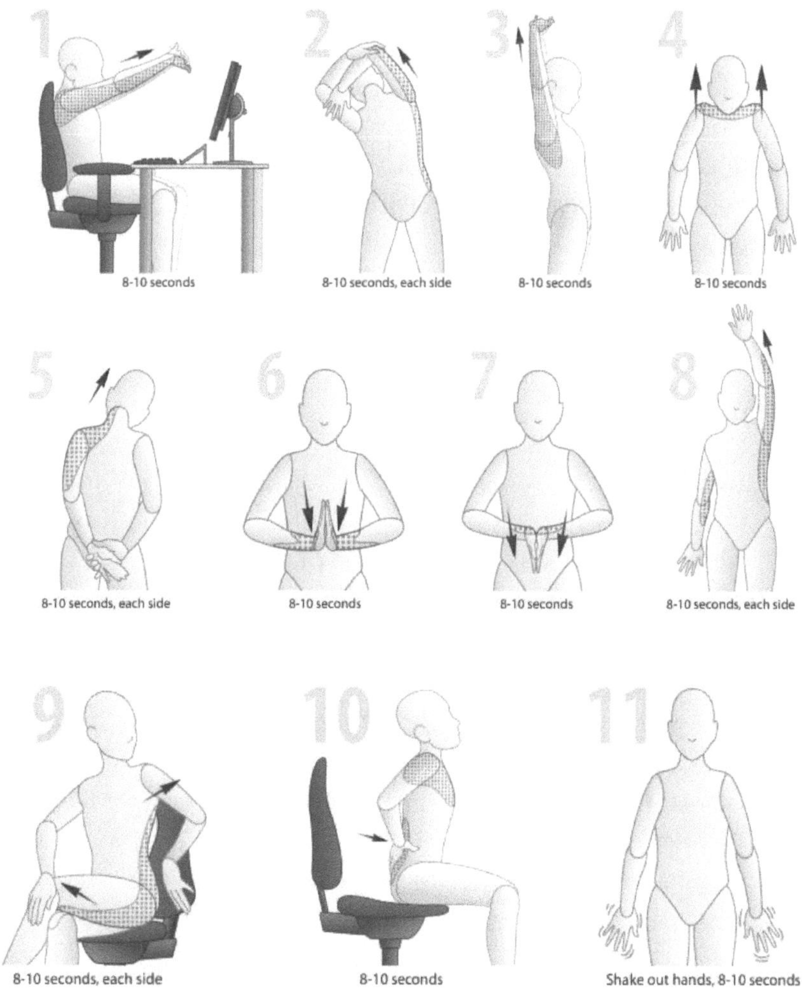

References:

1. OSHAnswersoftheCanadian CentreforOccupationalHealth andSafety(CCOHS) http://www.ccohs.ca/oshanswers/
2. OSHLinks:Ergonomicsof theCCOHS http://www.ccohs.ca/oshlinks/ subject/ergonomics.html
3. and Kuorinka T (Eds.). Ergonomic workplace analysis. Helsinki, Ergonomics Section, Finnish Institute of Occupational Health, 1997. ISBN:9518016747. [Available from bookshop at www.ttl.fi/internet/english)
4. Bridger RS. Introduction to Ergonomics, (2nd edition), and accompanying instructor's manual. Published by Taylor & Francis, 2003. ISBN 0-415-27378-1.
5. NOISH Lifting index and maternal handling technique.
6. Canadian Standards Association. (2017). Office ergonomics – An application standard for workplace ergonomics (CAN/CSA Standard No. Z412-17)
7. Read, G.J.M., Salmon, P.M., Goode, N., & Lenné, M.G. (2018). A sociotechnical design toolkit for bridging the gap between systems-based analyses and system design.*Human Factors and Ergonomics in Manufacturing & Service Industries*,*28*(6), 327-341.
8. Wilson, J. R. (2014). Fundamentals of systems of ergonomics/human factors. *Applied Ergonomics (45), 5-13.*
9. Hendrick, H. W. (2003). Determining the cost-benefits of ergonomics projects and factors that lead to their success. *Applied Ergonomics, 34,* 419-427.
10. OSHA Ergonomics eTool: Materials Handling: Heavy Lifting
11. OSHA Ergonomics eTool: Ergonomic Principles Index – Lifting
12. UCLA Ergonomics
13. Dul J, Neumann WP. Ergonomics contributions to company strategies. Applied ergonomics. 2009 Jul 1;40(4):745-52.
14. Pheasant S. Ergonomics, work and health. Macmillan International Higher Education; 1991 Oct 31.
15. Burov O. Human factors/ergonomics in eWorld: methodology, techniques and applications. InInternational Conference on Applied Human Factors and Ergonomics 2019 Jul 24 (pp. 459-464). Springer, Cham.

16. Harris C, Straker L. Survey of physical ergonomics issues associated with school childrens' use of laptop computers. International journal of industrial ergonomics. 2000 Sep 1;26(3):337-46.
17. Nichols S. Physical ergonomics of virtual environment use. Applied Ergonomics. 1999 Feb 1;30(1):79-90.
18. Hollnagel E. Cognitive ergonomics: it's all in the mind. Ergonomics. 1997 Oct 1;40(10):1170-82.
19. Long J, Whitefield A, editors. Cognitive ergonomics and human-computer interaction. Cambridge University Press; 1989 Jun 15.
20. Jørgensen AH. Thinking-aloud in user interface design: a method promoting cognitive ergonomics. Ergonomics. 1990 Apr 1;33(4):501-7.
21. Hendrick HW. Ergonomics in organizational design and management. Ergonomics. 1991 Jun 1;34(6):743-56.
22. Duffy VG. The impact of organizational ergonomics on work effectiveness: with special reference to concurrent engineering in manufacturing industries. Ergonomics. 1999 Apr 1;42(4):614-37.
23. Hendrick HW. Determining the cost–benefits of ergonomics projects and factors that lead to their success. Applied ergonomics. 2003 Sep 1;34(5):419-27.
24. Goggins RW, Spielholz P, Nothstein GL. Estimating the effectiveness of ergonomics interventions through case studies: Implications for predictive cost-benefit analysis. Journal of Safety Research. 2008 Jan 1;39(3):339-44.
25. Mike F, Patrick W and Colin M 2015 Macro and Micro Ergonomic Outcomes in Healthcare: Unravelling the Relationship between Patient Handling Performance and Safety Climate (Loughborough Design School: Loughborough University.
26. Panjaitan N, Ali AY. Clasification of ergonomics levels for research. InIOP Conference Series: Materials Science and Engineering 2019 May 1 (Vol. 505, No. 1, p. 012040). IOP Publishing.

FSC
www.fsc.org
MIX
Papier | Fördert gute Waldnutzung
FSC® C083411

Kolibri 360 GmbH
Ferdinand-Jühlke-Straße 7
99095 Erfurt, Deutschland
produktsicherheit@kolibri360.de

Druck:
CPI Druckdienstleistungen GmbH
im Auftrag der
Kolibri 360 GmbH
Ferdinand-Jühlke-Str. 7
99095 Erfurt